I0541649

GLINT

of

LIGHT

GLINT
of
LIGHT

23 End-of-Life Stories

CAROLYN
ROHRBACH

Copyright © 2023 Titania Lane

All rights reserved. This book or any portion thereof may
not be reproduced or used in any manner whatsoever
without the express written permission of the publisher
except for the use of brief quotations in a book review.

ISBN: 979-8-9879787-3-3 (Paperback)
ISBN: 979-8-9879787-1-9 (Hardcover)
ISBN: 979-8-9879787-2-6 (eBook)

Illustrations by Torunn Larsen

Book design by *the*BookDesigners
Cover image © Shutterstock

First printing, 2023

www.CarolynRohrbach.com

For my father-friend, Dick, and his white horse.

"Don't tell me the moon is shining; show me the glint of light on broken glass."

—*Anton Chekhov*

CONTENTS

MIDWIFING GRACE

I enter your home,
  in life's winter season.

My warm hand can hold
  many burdens.

My warm heart
  can bear witness to your suffering—
  and your courage.

Companioning the human spirit
  is not easy.

Not everyone is comfortable
  in the dark.

We are not always filled
  with grace.

But before I walk you home,
  let's sit here in the dark together.

I want to show you the stars.

1

SOCK MONKEY

As I drove to the board-and-care home that vivid morning, I thought about the life experiences and the people that had brought me to this work. Becoming a hospice spiritual counselor had been divine intervention. Then, knowing my past didn't belong in your present, I let my thoughts go.

As I walked into your room, the stark walls felt cold and forgotten. The closed window blinds offered little connection to anything outside. Dressed in a hospital gown, you lay on your side in a hospital bed, your long feminine shape covered by the neatly folded facility blanket. The surroundings offered little information about who—or what—was important to you.

I sat in the vacant metal chair at your bedside, offering gentle tones and soft whispers, not wanting to frighten you. Your frail hands clutched the stainless-steel bed rails as if you were afraid of falling. I decided it was best not to touch your hand or arm, though I did push the longer strands of hair away from your face. You never opened your eyes. You didn't let go of that bed rail either. I asked if I could return. Because you didn't speak or offer resistance, I took that as a "yes."

As weeks passed, you allowed me to rest my warm hand on yours. You silently clutched that bed rail all day and night as if it was keeping you from sinking. The endless grasp was wearing out the skin on your fingers and palms, and I wondered what your hands had been through, what they had held, and what they had let go.

When your son returned my phone call, I explained my role and my interest in bringing you comfort. He stoically reported on your life of mental and physical abuse. His voice more detached, he explained the generational cycle of abuse you shared with your own children. As your only son, he felt responsible for paying for your care but not for caring for you. I asked no follow-up questions. He had clearly worked hard on creating boundaries, and it was not my place to disrespect or push them.

The next time I sat in the frigid chair at your bedside, I asked you questions. *Who taught you about anger? Who taught you about betrayal? When did it start?* You didn't answer, but I held your hand again that afternoon.

Over the weekend when my own daughter cleaned out her closet, I got an idea. From her pile of once-loved stuffed animals, I pulled out a stuffed monkey—the kind with the bright red mouth made from an old woolen sock. Its long arms, legs, and tail were about the same size as your bed's rails you held on to so tightly. I smiled the following Tuesday when you took hold of that monkey's arm. I wanted the soft and warm to replace the hard and unforgiving. The sores on your palms seemed equally pleased with the change. You never let go of that monkey. It became threadbare from your clutched fists, but your palms seemed grateful. I think your heart was, too.

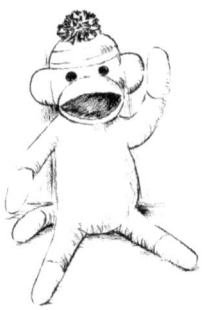

The unraveling was slow, but you began to leave your body. It was time. The transition took a week or two. Each day heat poured out of the crown of your head with such force your nurse, social worker, and I wondered how such a transition was possible. The heated tensions continued to radiate from the highest point of your head as we sat in awe of all that you carried. Bearing witness to the fervor, I held your clenched fists and tried to hold a sacred space. I wanted your feverish transition to result in alchemy.

You died on Christmas Eve. I like to think you had your own rebirth that holy night.

٠'،

In all my years of this work, I have never witnessed a more sustained and heated transition. Thank you for allowing me to witness your suffering. May your rage be replaced by the love you so deserved but never received.

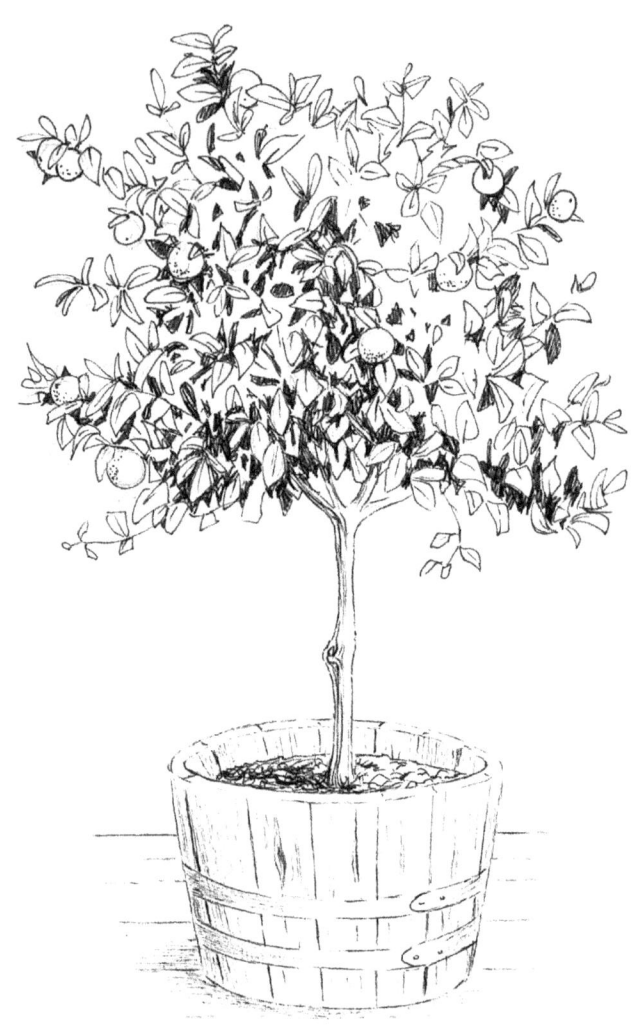

MS. ORANGE TREE

You answered the phone on the first ring.

"I'm a part of your hospice care team," I began. "You've already spoken with your nurse and social worker, but I'm your third team member, your spiritual counselor. It's a funny job title, but I'm here to see if you're in good spirits or poor spirits about coming onto hospice."

"I'm doing okay."

"Coming onto hospice can be a big decision," I added.

"Who are you again?" you asked, seemingly confused by so many recent calls from strangers.

"I'm a part of your hospice care team. The nurse helps with medications and your other physical needs. The social worker can help you get your affairs in order or help with any resources you might need. We all work closely together. The continuity of your care and how we support you is important to us. My role on the team isn't necessarily to be interested in what's happening with your body or your paperwork. I'm more interested in how you're doing on the inside. Not all pain is physical. We want to make sure you are well-supported physically, emotionally, and spiritually." I paused. "How are you feeling with all of these recent changes?"

"Okay, I guess. I don't think about it too much."

"Sometimes it can be helpful to talk with someone who has spent time with others on hospice. I would like to meet you and give you a face to go with my name. May I stop by tomorrow?"

"Are you from a church?" Your tone changed.

"No, I'm from hospice. You can be in good spirits or poor spirits with, or without, going to church, don't you think?"

"Yes, I just want to make sure you're not from a church." You sighed deeply.

"I am not, but if you would like to meet with

a minister, priest, or rabbi, I would be happy to arrange that."

"No, I don't want any of that."

"That's fine, but I'd rather ask and have you say 'no' than not ask and have it be something meaningful to you. Could I stop by tomorrow and introduce myself?"

"Sure." Then you hesitated with an audibly hard swallow. "Can I ask you a question?"

"Of course."

"Are you the one I'm supposed to die with?"

✦

The next day, I sat on the yellow loveseat in the tidy front room of your manufactured home. I answered your questions, assuring you there was no "right" or "wrong" way to die. Like many people with a terminal diagnosis, you seemed eager to talk about the details of dying. You wanted to know how it would work and what the norms and protocols were. You seemed concerned you would do the wrong thing or somehow make a social misstep at the end of your life.

"How am I supposed to do this? I don't want to screw it up," you said more than once.

I offered continued reassurances and encouraged you to think about what *you* wanted. *Where would* you *like to be? Who, if anyone, would you like near you?* I assured you I would visit often and answer as many questions as I could.

Over the next several months, I would learn how much you valued your independence. Your war-bride marriage had been an unhappy one, and you had learned from an early age to take care of yourself and not rely on others. You were kind and thoughtful but let very few people get close. You made it clear you wanted to die in your home, where you "belonged."

As your heart and lungs grew more fatigued, I watched you steady yourself with the furniture. From the armrest of the couch, you shifted to the end table, resting a moment before slowly turning to lean into a dining room chair. From there, you proceeded to the dining table. You scooted around the table to the credenza on the back wall, hanging on to something the whole way. Then you grabbed the doorknob that led to the kitchen and shuffled to the strategically placed bar stool a few feet from your kitchen counter. Your "furniture surfing" skills took their toll but agreeing to use a walker can be difficult for someone as independent as you were.

Your care team expressed concern over your "fall risk." We talked about technology and caregiving options that would allow you to stay in your own home as safely and independently as possible. You stoically refused to consider even the smallest changes.

The social worker and I asked what you thought might happen if you fell and injured yourself while you were alone.

"I would need someone to water my orange tree," you answered.

A bit frustrated with your unwillingness to protect yourself, I said, "Tell me more about your tree."

"Oh, it's a real beauty. I water it every day. I planted it in an old wine barrel I got from a neighbor. That tree keeps me moving. Some days it's the only reason I get out of bed. She needs her water."

I asked if I could see the tree, and you led me out your front door and down the two porch steps to the corner of your single-wide home to its place in the sun. It truly was one of the happiest trees I'd ever seen. Each full branch seemed to delight in offering its little round fruit. The tree held a special place in your heart, and I could see why.

On each visit after that, I always offered my *hellos* and *goodbyes* to your tree. It just seemed like the right thing to do.

Your death would come after a heated battle with your adult son. He made the long drive from his home after you took a nasty fall in the bathroom early one morning. He insisted you move into a care facility. You refused, and it got ugly.

The next day, and against your will, he physically moved you to a small board-and-care home on the other side of town. I knew you felt betrayed.

On your first afternoon in the facility, I walked down the long quiet hallway knowing you had landed right in the middle of your worst fear. I peeked around the corner of the door so as not to startle you. I gently asked if I could come in.

In my heart, I wanted to give you every bit of dignity, every bit of control that I could. With your permission, I sat on a dining room chair that had made its way into the room. Its gold upholstery was covered with a thick protective vinyl that made a displeasing sound when I sat on it. Then it was quiet, and you were withdrawn.

"I wanted to see you today," I said, still trying to let you lead.

You quietly asked for your purse. I stood and looked around but saw nothing personal in the space. You asked me to try a drawer. One drawer had a few nightgowns, the second, your purse.

I handed it to you, but you didn't make a move to receive it.

"My hairbrush is in there," you murmured without looking at me.

I hesitated, not because I didn't want to brush your hair, but because it was the first time you let me help. I sat beside you on the bed, carefully keeping you covered. You sat up, freeing your hair from the worn white pillow. I brushed the thick strands slowly and carefully with your wood-handled brush.

I knew the ritual of having your hair brushed must have been meaningful to you. The silent and repetitive action soothed you in some unknown way. As I worked my way to the other side, I gently asked, "Who else used to brush your hair?"

You took your time answering as if you were deciding whether you wanted to tell me. "My mother," you said softly, and I let it be.

In silence, I mindfully brushed every strand again. I brushed your hair till it shone like the sun on your beloved tree. I offered reassurances as to how amazing your hair looked, and you lay back down. I arranged the locks around your face and tidied the bedding back around you.

You folded your hands together and closed your eyes.

I returned to the noisy chair but didn't say anything. Several minutes passed. You opened one eye and looked at me.

"You're still here," I said, with a smile and half a laugh. Today, you didn't think I was funny. You closed the eye again and took a deep breath before exhaling. We sat in silence again.

In time, you opened the same eye. This time about half-mast. "Would you like me to leave?" I asked. You closed it again without responding. I didn't know whether to stay or go. Eventually, I said in a soft voice, "I don't know if I'm helping you or irritating you. I like sitting with you, but I don't know what you want."

You didn't answer. You didn't move.

Your cheeks were pink, your breathing was

relaxed and peaceful. Your brow was not furrowed, and your hands were resting gently. Your hair looked amazing.

I decided to leave and let you rest. I stood up but then second-guessed myself. I walked into the hallway and stopped, uncertain. I thought you might want space, but something didn't feel right. I leaned my back against the blank wall outside your room. I was facing you but no longer in your space. I held still. You opened the same eye.

"I'm still here," I called out. "Should I stay?" You didn't respond, just took another exasperated rhythmic breath.

I stayed, still again, in the unknowing.

A caregiver questioned my presence in the hallway, asking if I needed anything or if something was wrong. "I'm just not sure whether to stay or go." The caregiver encouraged me to leave because I had been there a while.

Loud enough so you could hear me, I instructed the caregiver to call hospice if you wanted me to return after your nap. She assured me she would. I said in an even louder voice, "I want her to know I'm here if she needs me."

I walked back to my car, still not knowing if I should be staying or going. I sat alone in my own space for a while and rolled the window down. A large crow settled in a tree just outside your window. "Will you hold the high watch for her?" I asked out loud. The crow didn't answer me, either.

An hour later, in the early evening, the caregiver checked on you, and you were gone.

\'/

I hope you found your peace, dear one. I hope you found your mother.

I just know she loved your hair.

SEASONAL VERANDAS

You sat in a white plastic patio chair on the concrete slab next to your one-room cinder block home. You were tan, with a jolly red face, genuine smile, white beard, and white shaggy windblown hair. You looked like Santa Claus on his post-Christmas tropical vacation. The plastic tubing from an oxygen concentrator snaked out your partially open front door, up and over the wall-mounted mailbox, and behind an empty planter box. After coiling on the cement, it nestled in your shaggy mustache just under your sun-tanned nose. It was obvious that both you and the oxygen tubing spent a lot of time outside in this very position.

"Are you my spiritual guru lady?" You chuckled. "Come join me here on my veranda." You pointed to a flimsy, sun-faded chair next to you.

I retrieved my sunglasses and accepted your offer.

"Lovely veranda you have here." I took in the view of your parking lot.

"This is my summer veranda," you clarified. "My winter veranda is over there." You pointed to the opposite edge of the worn concrete slab, nine feet directly behind us.

"Ah," I offered. "I will have to save that veranda for the holidays."

You laughed and clapped your hands like I was an old friend who'd been away for too long. I smiled at you and tilted my face toward the sun as we both enjoyed the sea air.

On and off for the next three years, you and I repeated this reception. As your sea-worn body continued the good fight, you improved enough to be discharged from hospice and admitted to the agency's palliative care program. Then you eventually declined again and returned to the hospice program. I was the only staff member to follow you between the two programs as your health ebbed and flowed.

Piece by piece, you told me your stories of being a young boy just outside Boston's great harbor. Even as a child, you were well-read on the ocean's navigation, history, and culture. Your fascination with the sea kept you out of trouble in the old Irish-Catholic neighborhood.

In your early twenties, you ignored your seagoing instincts and did what you were told to do. You got a "good job," married "a good Catholic girl." You had a half dozen kids and bought a house. You also became dangerously unhappy. For more than a decade, anger and alcohol anesthetized your pain. You left deep wounds on those around you. You knew your soul was out of alignment with the path you had chosen. When the pain could push you no further, the sea pulled you back, and you left the job, the house, the wife, and all six kids.

It might be easy to judge you for running away from the responsibilities you had willingly taken on. It might be easy to hear your story and jump to conclusions. But what if everyone dared to listen to their inner knowing? What if there were no expectations of family and nation? What would each of us do if we could hit the reset button? It is easy to judge but kinder to attempt understanding.

As I sat on your winter veranda, judgment-free, it was evident that you had lived joyous and sober on a boat longer than you had lived angry and drunk on land. Day after day, year after year, you were happy and content. You had what you needed and wanted nothing more. You had good friends and only a handful of regrets. You were open and honest about your choices. Even as your body declined, you continued to be curious. You continued to be free.

Three weeks before you died, in response to the wishes of your eldest son, you revoked hospice care to have a drain put into your chest. Your son criticized you for not exhausting every available medical option. Despite your own hospice wishes to focus on the comfort and quality of life, you agreed to a new treatment plan and hospitalization. Your attempted recovery in the hospital was long and fraught with setbacks. After ten days, they moved you to a reha- bilitation facility, but you never returned to your winter or summer verandas.

You died with a kind stranger holding your hand—a seasoned vocational nurse who had just started her shift. No memorial or boat parade was held in your honor.

I struggled with your death. Your hospice nurses and the social worker did, too. Along with your pal- liative care nurse, we decided to gather on our lunch break. We lit a candle, read a poem about the sea, and gave thanks for our three-year journey with you. One of the gifts of this work is being able to say goodbye. We get to see death come, and we get to sit with it for a while before letting each person go. We were sad you did not get to come home. We never got to say goodbye.

MALL RUN

We met the day before Thanksgiving. At twenty-three, you were one of my youngest patients. You loved showing off the happy scrapbook you worked so hard to create. Each sticker-framed page was full of photos documenting people celebrating.

Your bedroom's bright paint mirrored the colorful pillows and beanbag chairs that covered the floor. Every wall was filled with posters, mementos, fairy wings, and twinkle lights. The space itself seemed to be documenting a happy celebration, too.

You showed me your pile of completed Christmas cards and exquisitely wrapped gifts. You were eager for your Black-Friday-Mall-Run, an annual pilgrimage you completed with your mom. The overstuffed closet and mounted whiteboard shopping list made it clear retail therapy had been an important part of your treatment regimen.

You hugged me extra tight before I left. I remember because your long hug was in sharp contrast to our short and social conversation. Your thin frame melted into my arms as you pressed yourself against me. I squeezed back and asked if you were okay. You didn't answer, but you leaned into me again before releasing yourself and bounding back to your bed. I hesitated and wondered if should stay longer. You seemed to sense my thoughts and offered up an enthusiastic "Bye!" before I could offer.

Three days later, on Saturday, after all your new Black Friday purchases were wrapped and labeled, you died.

\'/

It might seem odd that I remember you so well. We had only spent an hour together.

It was your mother who left a mark on my heart. Not because she lost her daughter, but because she seemed to have lost everything else.

The house that held your room and the rest of your family was itself plain and stark. There were no flowers, no thoughtfully placed possessions, and certainly no celebratory pictures or fairy lights. The house, your dad, and your brother didn't look abandoned; they just felt forgotten.

I wondered what it was like for you to always be the target of your mother's laser-like focus. I wondered if she remembered that she had a husband and healthy son. I wondered if she ever remembered herself.

ᐩ

Being a caregiver can be a sacred act of love and companionship, but it can also provide the perfect hiding place from life. In the busy attentiveness we can distract ourselves from the feelings we don't want to feel. And yet, letting the urgent always crowd out the important has consequences.

\'/

When I think about your family, I am reminded to stop and look around. To notice who and what surrounds me every day. What support am I taking for granted or not seeing clearly? When I run around distracted all the time, my days feel incredibly long. You remind me that long days add up to very short years. I don't want to miss them.

HOSPITABLE TIRES

One of the things I love most about hospice work is its focus on comfort care, not treatment plans. Comfort is not only physical pain control, but about dignity and quality of life. The word "hospice" comes from the word "hospitality." Certain houses, or structures, along trade routes throughout Europe, became known for their entertainment, plentiful food, or medicinal knowledge. These "medical hostels" were the beginning of "hospice" as we know it today. Caring women with knowledge of herbs, oils, and other natural tinctures would skillfully try to ease the pain and suffering of the sick and the dying.

Throughout the Middle Ages, these hostels became the saving grace for the sick, hungry, and poor. Hospices de Beaune, in France, is one such place that is still standing. The compound is an ancient testament to humans caring for fellow humans. Its breathtaking Gothic structures from the early 1400s offer a glimpse into the world of ancient hospice wisdom and traditions.

The large main sick room, now historically staged, is lined with tiny beds divided by curtains in opulent red velvet to provide each occupant the luxury of privacy. All the flatware, plates and even bedpans were made from the finest metals, offering reverence and dignity to the ill and most disadvantaged.

I was fortunate enough to spend time walking the grounds and sitting in the room used for the actively dying. This sacred space was built on a bridge-like structure over a small river. A three-inch trench was carved into the floor so the dying would always hear the running river water below them. The room was also home to the only fireplace in the compound, except for the kitchen. There was no fireplace in the room for the sick or the staff. Only the dying were kept warm.

As I studied my new patient case notes that morning, I thought about the room in France, its grand hearth, open floor, and running river all created for the most impoverished. You were a challenging case for our staff. The police and a host of other elder-abuse services were already involved. As all the logistics were discussed, I wondered if anyone had held your hand. I thought of all the hospice workers over the centuries who had provided comfort and dignity in death to those who had received neither in life. I took a breath and offered a deep prayer of appreciation to those hospice workers who had come before me and on whose shoulders I was about to stand.

※

I found you on a single bare mattress with nothing but an old bath towel around you. The broken farmhouse where you had once lived and where you were now dying had no furniture and few intact windows. I could see the old floor, your mattress, and tires—stacks of tires. Some appeared brand new with chalk marks. Other, larger, tires had some miles on them. I don't know why you and the tires shared a space. I hoped it was that someone cared about you as much as they cared about their neatly stacked tires.

Besides stealing your hospice medications, your family member also seemed to be stealing tires. Your case was difficult to navigate, as the safety and comfort we wanted for you was not in alignment with your desire to "never leave family." Others—not I—were managing those concerns. My role was not to change your situation but to honor you in it.

I knelt beside you and dropped a shopping bag near your feet. I opened a water bottle and offered you a few needed sips, leaving a second bottle on the floor beside you. As I held your hand, I shared the history of hospice and the long traditions of caring for the sick. You looked at me while I spoke, making eye contact and squeezing my warm hand with your icy fingers. I wrapped the old bath towel tighter around your shoulders and unpacked my shopping bag.

With your permission, I gently rolled you from one side of your mattress to the other. I covered the stains with a cotton sheet. I removed the stained t-shirt you wore and replaced it with a soft flannel nightshirt. I smoothed your hair and wiped the dirt from your face. You knowingly blinked twice.

As I laid the clean cotton sheet over you and tucked the new blanket around your body, you melted into its soft warmth. I watched you sleep as I humbly offered a prayer of gratitude for you and for the lineage of hospice workers who lovingly honor all people, no matter how broken, disadvantaged, or mistreated.

I left a second shopping bag in the seemingly abandoned kitchen. I wanted to thank the person who cared enough to place you on a mattress.

＼'／

May we all allow one another to die with grace.

    May we all allow one another to die with dignity, especially those who have fallen.

MULTIPLE LIFE LADY

Days with blue skies and warm breezes make me think of our walks. The little flowers growing in the sidewalk cracks always brought you such joy. I'm still not sure if you looked forward to my weekly visits or just the walks around your neighborhood.

I will always remember you waiting for me in your garage. I'd pull up and there you were—sitting on the bench seat of your walker, shoes laced, wearing a light jacket and a big sun hat. Your enthusiasm was always contagious. We'd walk to the end of your street talking about the flowers and trees, which of course led to discussions of faith. I learned much from your deeply held beliefs of reincarnation and multiple lives. You were very well-read, and you seemed to enjoy sharing your wisdom with a captive audience.

We talked about your dementia diagnosis and

your long love of crochet. As the months passed and discussions deepened, our walks lengthened. The end of the street became a left turn and up a small hill. Soon we were walking around the block. Our team loved you so much that we didn't want to discharge you, but we all knew you were no longer declining. Before we graduated you from hospice, I hugged you. You told me I'd be back before you forgot about me. I laughed and silently hoped it was true. Eight months later your name appeared in my morning inbox. I was both sad and ecstatic.

Our walking days over, we sat on your patio and talked about the apple tree and flowers that brought you new joys. You remembered the feeling of walking with me, but details and words were now harder to find. Instead, the muscle memory of crochet became your happy place. Hour after hour, day after day, your fingers would glide the yarn back and forth over the hook. The routine comforted you.

During one of our visits, you handed me a crochet hook with a few rows of turquoise yarn already woven together. You were so disappointed when I shared my progress the following week, as your fingers quickly unraveled my work. I smiled as you replaced my stitches with your own.

Two more months passed, and your broken words were further unraveling. On a good day, just three weeks before you died, you looked me in the eyes and told me you wouldn't be able to remember me. You wanted me to know we would see each other again, though: "In Asia. We will be sisters." I hugged you tight and told you I loved you, too.

The following week, I sat quietly watching your busy fingers move the yarn back and forth... back and forth... as the Sinatra channel belted out one ballad after another. Your loving daughter was grateful for the quiet respite I provided her that afternoon.

The next visit we held hands as you slept in your favorite chair, covered in afghan squares stitched with love. Tony Bennett had replaced Sinatra, and even he was quieter.

I still hold guilt about your death. I loved you

so much and wanted to give you a "good send off."
I had been studying Celtic traditions and thought
it would be beautiful to anoint you before you
passed. I packed my oils and recited the words over
and over until I walked into your room that final
week. You slept as I enthusiastically told you about
my ritual. I knew right then you didn't like the idea,
but I did it anyway. I wanted the practice. I put my
own needs ahead of yours, and you deserved better.

As I drove away from your house that final day,
my small self said I'd honored you, but along the
freeway, I looked between the tall trees at the blue
sky and my deeper self corrected me.

My work that day had not been sacred. I had
served my ego instead of your spirit. The guilty
ache in my stomach assured me I would honor you
by never making that mistake again.

\'/

The crochet hook you gave me still sits on my shelf, a small piece of turquoise yarn still wrapped around it. I want you to know that if I could go back and do it again, I would just sit quietly at your bedside. I would hold your hand, and I would tell you I loved you—in this life and, maybe, even in the next one.

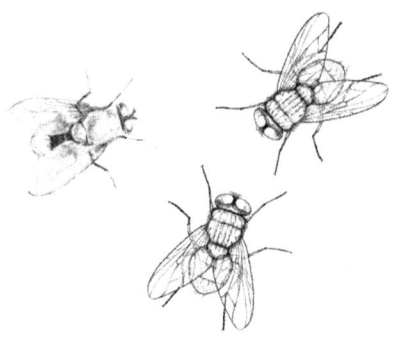

Fly Totem

When the fly arrives in your life it means something within you has changed. Let go of what is no longer serving you. It is time to be reborn into something new.

MY FLY GUY

Born the eleventh child of eleven children to an exhausted and depleted mother, you were cared for by your then nine-year-old brother. As your angry father gambled away the money on cock-fighting and alcohol, the family scattered. By the time you should have gone to school, nothing was left. You spent the rest of your life trying to reconcile your tragic start.

A drug gang provided much-needed food, shelter, and security—we all need that when we're ten years old. Those wounded boys and men taught you to anesthetize your pain through violence and drugs. You were a kid with no strategy and no opportunities. As you discovered through your life, pain that is not transformed is always transferred.

After thirty-plus years in federal prison for the unspeakable, I found you asleep on a previous girlfriend's couch. You looked peaceful, wrapped in blankets that had probably never been washed. The ashtrays were full, but the pill bottles were neatly arranged in a row. The Nature Channel was on. There was an unusual number of house flies in the small room you now called home.

I knelt on the dirty floor beside you and gently said your name. You didn't respond. I paused for a moment and studied the artwork decorating your arms. I was eager for you to wake up, as I knew you had stories to tell.

I tried again. No response. I was struck by how content you looked—curled up like a small child. The cancer raging inside you was numbed by the patchwork of medicated adhesive squares stuck up and down your arms. I tried again, "Hey, wake up."

When you opened your eyes, I was greeted with unexpected warmth. Your soulful brown eyes had a spark to them. You righted yourself and glanced at my hospice name badge. "Which one are you again?"

After a brief introduction, you quickly assumed I was a Christian chaplain. You shared your testimony. A prison missionary group had baptized you and offered forgiveness instead of needles. They also taught you to read.

For eight months we prayed together, you and me. You talked. I listened. I asked questions. You bravely answered them.

Eventually, you told me your stories.

We connected over nature and the rest of God's creations. Even your friends, the flies, were "from God." That's why you didn't kill them or even swat them away. You were now committed to doing no harm.

As your body sharply declined, deep fear from within you resurfaced. Terrified to die and be judged for a lifetime of poor and brutal choices, you wept.

I stayed close. There was nothing to say. There was nothing to do. This was your time to heal. It was a privilege to sit next to you. It was a privilege to hold your space. To me, you were a beautiful human broken by life. You were a little boy who just wanted to be held and loved. You were an even more broken man with a good heart and a beautiful mind.

On an early morning in March, our home health aide called me. She knew. She bathed you that morning and wrapped you in clean sheets. You were too weak to argue. I slid next to you on the couch and rested your head on my lap. I stroked your hair—just as I did when my own children were young and needed comfort.

As I thanked you for the stories and truths you chose to share, you coughed. I raised your depleted body in my arms hoping gravity would clear your throat. "It's okay. I got you," I said.

You swallowed hard.

Your breath was shallow and had lost its rhythm. You gurgled a little, and I pulled you close. My eyes welled. You would not die alone. You sat up straight, releasing my arms. Your eyes popped wide open, and just like that, you were gone.

I felt you leave.

You were in a hurry, and I didn't blame you. I stayed there with you for a while.

And even the flies were quiet.

When the nurse arrived, I left you. You were in good hands. I walked back to my car, closed the door, and sobbed. Not because you were gone but because you never really got to live. You never got to love.

༈

I went home early that day. I would not be emotionally ready for another visit.

I took a shower. As the hot water soothed me, I felt you being held by God. He was washing your body and bathing you in light.

But if we walk in the light, as he is in the light, we have fellowship with one another, and the blood of Jesus, his Son, cleanses us from all sin. —JOHN 1:7

You would have liked that one.

LAVENDER LADY

I don't remember how long you had been in the facility when I met you, but you seemed content. Your body was nimble and fairly able, but your mind wasn't keeping up. I don't know what your last words were, or what you wished you could say. I never heard you make a sound.

Some advanced dementia patients felt like shells to me. Their bodies are there, but their spirits tend to come and go. It feels like they are in the here and now for a bit, but then they slip away for hours or even days before returning. But not you. You had a real presence. Your spirit didn't seem to roam.

Each day you sat in the large, multipurpose room in a nice wooden rocking chair. You were always dressed for the day with neat hair and a cheery quilt in your lap. Gently rocking yourself in front of the tall bookcase full of board games and books, you watched the hubbub—attentive staff talking, preparing snacks and meals, and assisting other residents. Occasionally a musician or children's choir visited. Without uttering a word, you watched it all.

Your attentive daughter visited daily. She had carefully decorated your room with past and present family photos. Well-made comfortable clothing filled your closet. She also boasted about your holiday traditions and homemaking skills. Her childhood home had been a gathering spot for neighbors, church groups, and a wide circle of friends. I was sorry to hear your husband had left when the children were grown. He quickly remarried, but you never did.

I listened carefully as your daughter eagerly shared stories from your life and hers. Paying attention to the stories of your life gave me important clues for what might bring you peace toward the end of it.

When I saw you next, I brought a teddy bear. Your roommate held a special doll as if it were her own child. I thought you might enjoy your own special treasure, but you had no interest.

In time I brought headphones with an attached microphone, wondering if by amplifying my voice in the noisy room you might enjoy a song or short reading. A human voice focused solely on you didn't interest you either.

Knowing that your children adored you, I imagined they sat on your lap as you read book after book to them in their youth. I tried brightly colored ones: *Goodnight Moon*, *Ferdinand*, and *Johnny Crow's Garden*. I read them to you with such gusto that two ladies on the corner couch were highly entertained, but you were withdrawn. I kept reading anyway.

I thought of you often between our visits. I challenged myself to get creative. How could I connect with you? If sight, sound, and touch weren't interesting, I wondered if smell would be.

The following week I pulled up my usual chair in front of you. Our knees almost touched as you held my gaze. At the start of each visit, we looked directly into each other's eyes. I was always the first to blink, but I saw you, and it felt like you saw me, too. After our greeting, I put three small bottles of oil on the side table—eucalyptus, lavender, and ginger. The scent of lavender caught you, your eyes twinkling. I smiled for you.

Before our next visit, I mixed grapeseed oil with a few drops of lavender and slipped the bottle into my bag beside the children's books, headphones, devotionals, and mouth swabs.

Every visit after that, we held each other's gaze as I spoke in gentle tones. I carefully opened the bottle under your watchful eyes and let the aroma linger under your nose. I gently rubbed the oil on your fingers, palms, and wrists, warming us both. It was a human connection: sight, sound, smell, and touch.

As time passed, your rocking-chair days ended. The quiet of your room, under that big window, became your sanctuary. Like your mind, your body was now fading. I sat at your bedside offering gratitude for our time together and for the afternoon sun that bathed you. As you started to spend time a little bit here, and a little bit somewhere else, I dabbed the inside of your wrists with our oil. I wanted to send you off with the best perfume friendship could buy.

You died a few days later, your favorite caregiver by your side.

٠'،

After meeting you, I always kept little bottles of oil in my bag. Not just for anointing the sick and the sad, but for honoring the connections we make to the world around us through our senses.

You, dear one, will always be my Lavender Lady.

AMPLIFIED PAIN

Seeing another human being in pain is never easy. The clenched jaw and tense muscles brace themselves for the next agonizing stab. It can be extraordinarily hurtful for both the victim and the observer.

Palliative (or comfort care) medicine, like the rest of the medical world, has improved greatly since Elisabeth Kubler-Ross first testified to the U.S. Senate about hospice pain management in 1972. Today, very few, if any, hospice patients die with uncontrolled physical pain.

Unless, of course, they want to.

⋎

The staff in your tiny board-and-care were surprised when I asked to see you. "He does not talk," the woman said in heavily accented English.

"He doesn't talk, or he can't talk?" I asked.

Both your nurse and case manager had told me to tread lightly. You had refused all comfort medications, social work, spiritual care, and every available support. I'm sure you would have refused the hospice nurse if her presence were not required by law. We all knew you only agreed to hospice care to avoid another 911 call made by the staff. You were done with hospitals.

When I entered your room, you lay on your side, facing the wall. Your back was to the room and to all those who might enter. I sat on the brown vinyl chair against the wall and sank into its thick foam seat. The chair reminded me of a bowling alley, and I wondered if it had come from the now-abandoned alley a few blocks over in this industrial side of town.

My feet firmly on the floor, I felt the weight of my body being supported by the bowling-alley brown. I did not place my warm hand on your cold shoulder. I chose instead to practice "companion breathing," matching the pace of my breathing with yours, breath for breath. It was quiet and peaceful in the room.

The following week, you faced the wall, your legs curled up—not quite knees to chest. I sat in the bowling-alley chair, pressed my back into the foam, my feet flat on the floor, and found my breath. Then I found yours. We repeated this ritual for weeks. I never asked you to speak or be anything different than you were. All I did was sit with you, fully present, your breath leading the way.

We knew nothing about you. No family listed. No personal information. Nothing personal in your room or on your bed. There was only a fiduciary agent who seemingly never returned phone calls.

Your skin started to break down from remaining in the same wall-facing position week after week. The staff reported your intense pain with every attempt to keep you clean.

You refused the special mattress to ease your skin. You refused every pain and comfort measure offered. Occasionally you opened your mouth for a sip of water or broth. Your physical pain became so intense that it was daunting for the staff to be with you.

We had the tools and skills to make this better. We had creams, ointments, patches, and pills. We had IVs, mattresses, and compresses. We had warm hands, kindness, and compassion. We could listen. We could have eased your suffering.

Or could we?

The last time I saw you, your face grimaced with each breath. Your whole body rigid, you were pressing your lips together with such force they were almost purple. Your eyes were squinted tight from the waves of burning nerve pain, and your breath was shallow for fear of expanding your lungs.

I returned to the brown chair, trying to hold the space for you to feel the pain and to want the suffering. It was difficult for me to bear witness to your stoic resistance. Before I left, I spoke: "May I ask why you want the pain?"

Your eyes opened suddenly. Through clenched teeth and shaking muscles, you glared at me. "I deserve this. I must suffer. *Now leave me alone!*" Your words were spewed with such venom and conviction that I knew there would be no other way out for you. This was your penance. Your hell.

I stood up and distanced myself but remained in your room.

Now I understood. All the compassion, concern, and kindness offered to you only added to your spiritual and physical pain. The more we tried to soothe and relieve you, the more you retreated. You wanted to fight, to suffer, to experience the hell you "deserved."

᭐

It is not for me to say whether your pain and suffering were warranted. That is God's business, not mine. But years later, I remember you. I remember your courage. You wanted to feel every ounce of the pain. On some level, it was your way of making amends. I'll never know if or how you hurt people. I'll never know if you found your peace.

What I do know is that you died the way you wanted to die and to me, that's the most important part. You felt it all.

BASS FISHERMAN

In early December, a month before you died, I returned to your tiny, subsidized apartment. Every week we visited, but this day was unique. I was excited for you as I wandered through the labyrinth of cement paths leading to your building and then to your door. I knocked and then pushed your door wide open.

"Let me see," I said, entering the sparse studio.

You lifted your head and smiled, almost in slow motion. You were slouched in your wheelchair, swollen legs the size of tree trunks, eyes bright, with a smile that transformed your whole face. Your heart of gold was worn out, but your spirit was strong.

"I feel like a king," you said as I knelt beside you and leaned in. I wanted you to use your energy for the words, not the volume.

"This is my new table." You paused, again saving breaths for more sentences.

I studied the table's four-foot, rectangular, gray plastic top.

"The legs fold up inside the table, so you can put it away if you want," you added.

I ran my hand down one of its round black metal legs.

You pressed your hand on the top of the table's smooth, clean plastic. "It's pretty neat." You exhaled, turning your head away from the new treasure to look at me.

I knew it was the first brand-new, out-of-the-box table you had ever owned. Matching your pride, I responded, "It is really, really neat."

Then, starting from your left, you pointed to each new appliance. The coffee maker made six cups at once. You explained the different settings, the timer, and the computer chip inside. You said you didn't know when you'd make your first cup. You said it was too neat to use; you just wanted to look at it.

You took a few more sips of oxygen before commenting on the toaster oven. You liked it because it resembled one you'd had before. The tempered glass door still had its sticky peel-off glass protector.

Then came the air popper. You almost chuckled explaining how it worked, popping the kernels without oil. "Can you believe it? Technology!" you said, shaking your head.

The last in this grand row was an electric shaver. Unlike the others, it was still neatly tucked away in its box. You were less enthusiastic about this gadget, but it still had its place in the lineup.

I was genuinely excited for you. "How do you feel?" I asked moving over to the folding chair, my knees aching from the floor.

You looked at me, resting your chin in the palm of your hand to support the weight of your head, your elbows balancing on the arms of your wheelchair. "I never would have believed it," you said. "Who would have thought I'd ever live like a king?"

I offered a seated bow, as any commoner would do in the presence of royalty.

We both sat there for a while looking at the first brand-new appliances you had ever owned. You kept shaking your head as you pointed out more settings and features. It was your very own Christmas miracle.

You had spent most of your life doing concrete foundation work. Your broken body and exhausted heart reflected a lifetime of hard work in the sun. You'd rejected the unions on principle, you said, and had only received one week of paid vacation in your entire life. You had shared that meaningful story when I asked what you were most proud of.

We had visited each week for five and half months before you died in January. Our time together gifted me with a deep joy of human connection. Your smile filled my heart.

We had a few mishaps. More than once I found you on the floor in need of personal assistance when your failing heart didn't allow you to make it to the bathroom in time. You were so embarrassed but grateful for the help.

You wanted your hair cut before you died, so I pushed your wheelchair all the way to the barbershop. You yelled, "Faster, faster," as the wind pushed your shaggy strands away from your bright eyes. We laughed all the way back as the breeze tickled your newly exposed ears.

You were brave enough to share the darkness: difficult memories of your alcoholic father, your frightened mother, and your younger brother's death. We talked a lot about the highs and lows of living in a camp trailer for most of your life. You smiled as you talked about all the nights you fished for your own largemouth bass dinner. Interwoven into your dark feelings and memories was a great love of nature and the art of observation. You noticed things. You paid attention.

I don't think you ever married, and you never spoke of any great loves. You kept to yourself, never asking or wanting much. The social worker had helped you organize some paperwork, and you received a check for money owed to you. A hospice volunteer had taken you on a shopping spree and encouraged you to splurge. That was the day you brought home the treasured appliances you proudly showed me. It was a grand day.

You never did use those appliances.

\',

You died a wealthy man, my friend, not because of your new acquisitions or your newfound hospice friendships, but because of the gold in your old worn-out heart. I will forever treasure your smile.

THE ONE

When you choose to do this work—or maybe the work chooses you—there are always concerns regarding professional boundaries. It is sometimes difficult to navigate the written—and unwritten— rules of how to engage with people in one of the most intimate times of their lives, without getting too close, without getting too attached, without letting them in. It takes practice and discipline to find the balance of caring and companioning without getting personally involved.

If—or should I say *when*—you give too much of yourself, you can "burn out." The burden of grief, of death, of constantly loving and losing can become too much. How do you learn to start your workday each morning by opening your email to see who has died since you logged off? There is nothing worse than calling to schedule a visit when you are unaware that your patient has died hours beforehand.

There are rules in hospice care. You can call, text, and email but never from your personal phone or personal email address. This rule ensures patient privacy, but it also fortifies professional boundaries. Establishing healthy work habits can be challenging when people don't always die Monday through Friday from 8:00-5:00. People die on holidays, on weekends, and right in the middle of your week-long Hawaiian vacation. Death doesn't fit neatly into a predetermined schedule and time slot.

You can cry on the job, but you can never cry harder than the family. You can sit with someone for hours every week, for a year or two at a time, and know almost everything about them. You know their family dynamics and addictions, their regrets, and their fears. You can learn intimate details of their most significant accomplishments and of their deepest secrets. You can know their shame. And yet, they will never know any of yours.

Redirecting conversation back to the patient, to the family, and the matter at hand becomes a well-honed skill. I learned early on that I wasn't learning anything if I was the one talking. Being fully present and listening attentively was the medicine I could administer. Asking the right question at the right time is the holy grail of being a hospice spiritual counselor. Every day, with every verbal patient, it is the ultimate goal.

And then I met Charlene.

That is her real name. I use it here because I am still friends with her family, and I have their blessing. She was the first and only patient I let slip in, pull up a chair, and make herself at home right inside my professionally walled-off heart. Sure, I have loved others, some deeply, but Charlene made her way to my core.

In fairness to me, she was an extremely gifted therapist, with a long pedigree and a successful career. From day one, I was out-classed and out-skilled in every way. She became *my* mentor in life and in her death.

During each visit, I sat on her ottoman. She sat in her chair, surrounded by papers, a phone, mail, and books—everything she needed for the day always within arm's reach. My education and skills were no match for this seasoned professional who skillfully mentored me through the twists and turns of companioning.

We had spirited discussions about religion, faith, empathy, sacraments, premonitions, and hallucinations. We debated the nuances of "being a Christian" or embracing Christ's philosophies as a non-religious person, still seeking divine connection.

She was a master in the art of spiritual discernment. She led by example, and I willingly followed her right into my own deepest truths.

She believed in me. She had faith that I could do this work, that I *should* be doing this work. She encouraged me and corrected me when I crossed a line. Right up until her death, she mentored me and pushed me out of my professional comfort zone.

Even after she died, on the really hard days with a difficult death or challenging, complex visit, I drove by her house just to feel close to her. I sat in my car and saw her plants still potted on the front porch. I stared at her front door and knew I was never truly alone in this work.

Her death remains one of my favorites.

She had purchased a new dress for the occasion. She had tried it on to make sure she liked it and that it would be "comfortable." She talked about all the aspects of her life, her accomplishments, and her disappointments. In the same open and honest way, she sometimes questioned her faith and her fears. She made amends and made difficult phone calls. She wrote letters and cards to those she loved and to those she didn't. She cried, she grieved, she celebrated, and she felt sorry for herself. All of it was real.

As she lay in her bed, actively dying, her beloved niece was by her side. Her best friend arrived, then I arrived and joined the circle. I was the newcomer, having only been able to love her for ten short months.

We held hands around her. We lit candles. We took turns telling her how much we loved her. We shared what we would miss and laughed about the parts we hoped she would leave behind. We held still and collectively held her in our grace.

When she left our circle, we cried. We said a prayer and anointed her body. We bathed her in oils and dressed her in the new "comfortable dress." We wrapped her in the afghan she had stitched, combed her hair, and adorned her lips with pink. We folded her hands and sprinkled her with petals and rosewater. We celebrated the light and the love of our spiritual sister.

Friends and family came to her bedside to say their goodbyes and pay their respects. For three days, a vigil was held. For three days, there was a community in grief and in faith. It was a holy testimonial.

Charlene was cremated. Her family asked if I would pick her up. I willingly retrieved the black box with the brass tag and brought her home—to my house. I placed her on a table, looking out my biggest, brightest window. I shared her with my children. For several months she was an honored guest until her family came to take her home.

☼

Charlene has been gone a long time now, but her wisdom still lives inside me. Her picture sits on my shelf, and some of her books are in my bookcase. In a way, I continue to surround myself with her. She is the one I will never let go.

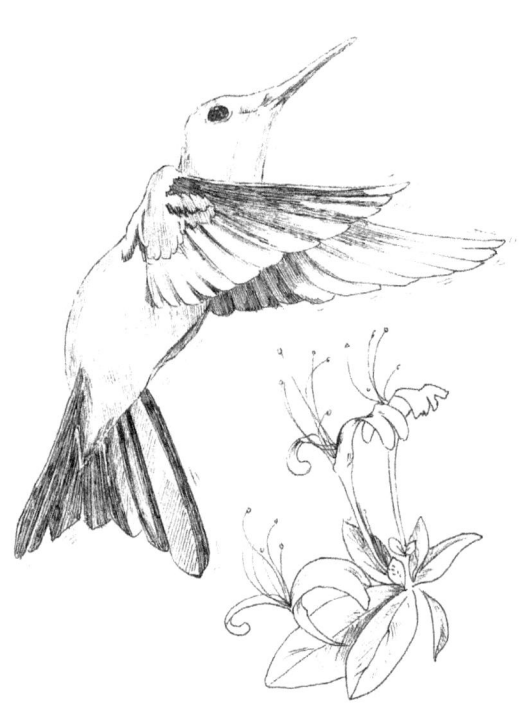

HUMMINGBIRDS

It is said that hummingbirds are a gentle reminder to always seek out the good in life. Your home was filled with these tiny, winged creatures on collectibles, stained glass suncatchers, and tea towels. Neatly stitched hummingbird pillows lined the couch and sat on each chair. You even had a hummingbird blanket on your bed.

You were tiny yourself. Like a happy hummingbird, you flitted from one topic to the next, engaging, asking, and sharing your thoughts and stories. Every afternoon you sat in your favorite chair next to your favorite window and listened to Wayne Dyer read his book from your abundant CD collection. You lit up talking about him, like a young schoolgirl talking about her first crush.

If Wayne Dyer was your crush, Lao Tzu was your father. You loved and respected him, always looking for his wisdom and guidance. You kept his picture in your pocket, pulling it out several times a day as if needing his assurance. Before you went to sleep each night, you pulled the picture from your pocket, kissed his face, and thanked him for protecting you. Then you carefully placed the photo on your nightstand.

You never expressed any fear of death. Your childlike wonder made death seem like a great adventure. You talked about it with anticipation and wonder, almost like it was a vacation. You often giggled in delight.

Then your daughter came to visit.

She shared a very different story of your life and childlike wonder. Her loving concern was that you would die with unfinished business in your heart. The events that took place when you were just fourteen years old seemed to have frozen you in time. Your daughter worried about the spiritual pain buried deep in your bones. It was a story you never told and didn't ask for. It was a story only others felt the need to share. More than seventy years after it happened, in the last year of your life, the story was again being told—this time to me.

When you were ready and in your own way, you were brave enough to speak it out loud. Together we held the space for it. The unburdening was slow at first, with the facts and events taking the lead, but then something shifted. We held still. There in your dimly lit bedroom the wounded inner child emerged and shared her story. I stayed silent knowing the divine was at work. Your daughter was right. All of you needed to be heard in order to be free.

The details of your story are not for me to share. You asked me to keep it safe, and I will. I do wonder if perhaps like the hummingbirds you surrounded yourself with, all you ever really wanted to do was fly backward and quickly change life's direction.

٧,

Sometimes in this work, as in life, stories are told. Terrible things happen. Some wounds heal and become scars. Other wounds fester for a lifetime behind fortified inner walls. When I think about you, I am reminded of my own burdens and joys. You remind me to sit outside near my honeysuckle bush so the hummingbirds can witness my story, too.

MRS. BEACH

Before walking up to your front door, I paused for a few moments. It had been a long day, and you were my last visit. I walked slowly, mindfully bringing myself to the present. I saw the yard, the house, and then the front porch. All of it was immaculate.

I rang the bell.

The front door swung open. I was greeted by a raised, terse voice. "Is Jesus Christ your Savior?" I hesitated, trying to stay focused. I wasn't sure if it was the unexpected tone of voice, the question itself, or your presence in the wheelchair that startled me. It was probably all of it.

"Well, *is* Jesus Christ your Savior? You can't come in here unless you are a Christian woman."

I offered the standard hospice answer: "I'm a hospice spiritual counselor. I meet with patients and families from all faith backgrounds. If you would like to meet with a Christian minister, I'm happy to arrange that for you, but I wanted to introduce myself. I work with your husband's nurse and social worker. I'm the third member of his care team."

"Is Christ your personal Savior and Lord?"

I steadied myself, willing my fatigue aside, and answered as honestly as I could. "I love Jesus' teachings. And I am a non-denominational part of your husband's care team."

Slam.

Exhaling, I took a few steps off the porch and stood there. No one had ever slammed a door in my face before. I walked back to my car and leaned against the hood. It would have been easier to drive away, but in my heart, I recognized the anger, control, grief, and fear of depletion. I had been there.

I slowly walked back up the path and tapped on the door, hoping it would be less intrusive than the first loud, jarring bell.

A meticulously appointed caregiver answered this time. I introduced myself as part of the team and asked if I could quietly visit the patient without disturbing you. She escorted me to the bedroom and left me alone with your sleeping husband. Clean and comfortable, he was slumbering deeply. I chose not to disturb him. I stood at his bedside as there was no chair and sitting on the bed felt too intrusive.

The tidy bedroom had a lot to say. You had married your handsome midshipman very young. He had achieved rank and status as you raised two children on military bases in faraway places. You now had grandchildren who looked neat as pins smiling up from sterling frames. Everything was in order, and everything had a place.

Except for that hospital bed.

And the Hoyer lift.

And the bedside commode.

The medical supplies and adult diapers disrupted the coordinating fabrics and trims. Your husband's failing mind and body, along with your own stroke-induced challenges, could not be organized, decorated, or disinfected.

I did not want to overstay my questionable welcome, so I walked along the outer edges of the vacuum lines on the deep carpet. It was not my place to disrupt the order of things. Projecting my voice, I thanked the caregiver, hoping you would hear me as well. I praised her for the immaculate care of the patient and home.

The following week I called, asking only about you. Acknowledging your church family and the abundance of food, flowers, and well wishes, I offered something I didn't think you had—privacy. I shared how other caring spouses often benefited from a safe person to talk with outside their usual circle of family and church friends. "I've been blessed to do this work for a long time," I shared. "I would be happy to support you in all of this. I can tell your husband is already very well taken care of." You reluctantly agreed, although truth be told, I don't think you knew I was the same person you'd slammed the door on.

For the next two months, we talked about the Bible and read scripture. You reviewed the well-executed life the two of you had built. Like the evenly spaced annuals lining your driveway, and the dust-free worldly treasures that lined your living room, all the achievements made sense. The 1960s woman who strived to be the perfect military wife and mother with the perfect faith had never expected to find herself weakened and wheelchair dependent. You also never expected to have a bedbound husband who no longer recognized you. The loss of independence and self-worth must have been crushing.

I asked about being married to an officer moving his way up the military hierarchy decade after decade. I asked about protocols, the wives' club, and moving from base to base with young children in tow. Some days you were more forthcoming than others.

In time, I asked how you took care of your own spirit. What was the space where you felt free? Was it in books? Baking? Music? The arts? You knew immediately what I was asking, and you didn't quote the Bible. Instead, you opened your heart just enough and told me about the beach. The way your father taught you to dig for clams, the way your children built elaborate sandcastles with moats.

A few weeks before your husband passed, you asked if I would take you to the beach a few miles from your home. After you swore your caregiver to secrecy, I broke with strict hospice protocol and took you. (Occasionally, a spiritual counselor must report to an even higher power.) You told me where to go, where to park, and how to maneuver the wheelchair up and over the low point in the boardwalk. It was apparent you had made this same trip many times over. You had planned every step of the escape.

I obeyed as I pushed you along the wooden pathway. We let the sun fall on our faces as the salt air freed us both from our burdens. We laughed into the wind.

You told me to push you out onto the packed sand. Against my better judgment, I did. I knew it would be hard work pushing you back, but it felt important. You wanted me to leave you alone. Again, overriding my voice of reason, I walked about ten yards back to the boardwalk and sat down out of your line of sight. For several uninterrupted minutes, I watched you watching the waves.

Then I saw you do it. I watched it happen.

You swung your head backward, then quickly thrust it forward. With just enough momentum, gravity tossed you out of that God-forsaken wheelchair and onto the sand. You log-rolled yourself about six feet before some good Samaritans came running. I leaped up, trying to get to you first. Running in the sand was not easy, nor was yelling at the top of my lungs into the wind. I ran past you, assuring the handful of helpful people that you were okay. I was with you. I did my best to safeguard your space as you flung the sand and screamed with your stroke-broken voice. The exhaustion and disillusionment from a lifetime of "being good" had taken their toll. For eighty-five years, you had come to the beach. Now, it was the only thing that could hold you.

The onlookers continued to be concerned as you cried, righting yourself with only one working arm.

I stood close, facing away, letting you be. I offered reassurances to well-meaning people. It's easy for humans to assume that all pain is physical. Only the sand and sea could hold your spiritual pain that day. Even your bones seemed to sink into the beach as if you were willing your broken frame to descend below the surface and escape like a clam.

You didn't say a word when I returned your spent body back to its wheelchair. You closed your eyes and remained silent on the drive back home. The caregiver was waiting at the curb.

The following week you wanted to take me "for a hamburger." I hesitated, knowing I could not continue to break you free. You thought it was necessary to "pay me back" for taking you to the beach, so you insisted. Mid-burger, I was about to tell you this would be our last outing, but you unintentionally knocked over your soda, loudly spilling it onto the tiled floor. You were embarrassed and started shaking. There was hardly anyone around, but I knew you felt humiliated by your inability to control your body. I tried to lighten the mood by tipping my soda over a bit and reassuring you that accidents happen. I felt helpless sitting across from you that day, watching your heart slam shut again.

You were polite during my next few visits, but our conversations were back to Bible study and social pleasantries. I pushed a little, trying to open the door again. You stoically declined, and I continued to respect your unspoken wishes.

Thirty days after our beach outing, your husband of more than sixty years died alone in his sleep during his afternoon nap. You were sitting at the kitchen table.

I saw you in the receiving line at his well-attended full-military funeral. You avoided my eyes and barely shook my hand.

٧,

Two weeks after your husband's service, your name appeared in my new-patient inbox. You had collapsed leaving the funeral, and your son had driven you to the emergency room. Your adult children assumed you were dehydrated and exhausted. It wasn't until the hospital admitted you that they learned of your prior cancer diagnosis. From the beginning, you had refused all treatment and told no one. Apparently, your caregiver kept lots of secrets.

I sat with you three times in your immaculate home before you died.

The first time, you were withdrawn, your daughter and caregiver lovingly at your side.

The second time, I sat quietly alone at your bedside. I wondered if the final physical loss of your husband made coming back to this house, this room, too painful. Had you planned your collapse? Had you planned to die in the hospital, never having to return home without him? Were you willing yourself to die? I held your hand. You seemed too exhausted to withdraw it.

The third time I saw you, I went to the beach first and sat on the sand where you tried to make your peace. When I returned to your bedside, you barely opened your eyes to look at me. As the same well-appointed caregiver straightened your pillows, your daughter was on the phone doing her best to keep things in order. I asked if I could spend some quiet time with you, and they didn't mind.

I sat with you a while and then stood up and carefully untucked the crisp hospital corners from your bed. I pulled the top sheet up and away, exposing your narrow feet and thin shins. Then I emptied my pockets. I smiled at the mess as the little grains of cold, dry sand sprinkled down on your toes, ankles, and fresh sheets, and I tossed a little more on your legs for good measure.

Proud of my work, I re-creased the hospital corners and re-straightened your blankets. I returned to your bedside, touched your hand, and gently whispered in your ear, "Did you think I was going to let you go without sand between your toes?" The corners of your mouth edged up a little, and I squeezed your hand before saying my goodbyes.

✶

Twelve hours later, just after three o'clock in the morning, as the waxing moon made its way over the sand and across the sea, you escaped.

THE DANCE

We met in the fall, just as the summer fog was clearing and the monarch butterflies were returning from the North. Your home, just blocks from the beach, had been your epicenter for over fifty years. You raised your family here. Your wife, the mother of your children, fought her cancer in this house and then died in your bed. You battled your own demons of grief within these walls. Many years later, a special girlfriend died in this house too.

Your home was the center point of your shrinking world. Like your own fine-tuned orchestra, your son, daughter-in-law, grown grandchildren, neighbors, friends, meal volunteers, and hospice staff all came by on their given days in their allocated time slots. Your family was desperate to keep you home. All you wanted to do was die in your own bed.

From the time you woke in the morning and made your slow heroic pilgrimage down the hall to the chair in the living room until you stoically returned to your bed each night, someone accompanied you. Each day, there was a never-ending trail of in and out, in and out, checking, doing, and adjusting to the world around you. My day was Tuesday, my time slot 1:00. I did not make your food. I did not adjust your oxygen or medications. I did not want to know when you went to the bathroom. I didn't care about your intake or your output. I had no interest in your swollen legs or your laundry. I sat in the repositioned kitchen chair directly across from your tan corduroy recliner and listened.

With great humor and a real zest for storytelling, you shared your military service stories between sips of oxygen. More than once, you told me about your security detail at the armed services psychiatric hospital. You recalled the antics of drunken sailors fighting in parking lots and late-night admissions into the military psych ward as if they'd happened yesterday. But the memories that made your whole face light up were the USO dances. On Saturday nights, you listened as the military band played their swing music. You played Ping-Pong, darts, and miniature bowling. Seventy years later, sitting across from me, you named the hostesses and described their perfumes. You longed to twirl them around the dance floor again.

About two weeks before you died, you did your best to say goodbye. We were both tearful. You were sleeping more than you were awake, and your legs could no longer carry you to the living room. I held your hand and repeated some of your stories to you, assuring you they would not be forgotten. We talked about your worn-out body and thanked it for its eighty-eight years of good service.

"Any regrets?" I said, smiling, already knowing what you would answer.

"I would've asked more girls to dance," you half-mouthed, half-whispered.

I smiled as I tucked you into your own bed.

٭

I ate my lunch on your front porch a few times after you died. I liked it there. I guess it was my way of saving you a dance.

THE WOMAN
WHO LOVED THE SKY

For two years and two months, I walked to your apartment, and this sign greeted me:

Live Well
Laugh Often
Love Much

Some days it was my own much-needed reminder; on others, it just made me smile. I knew the next hour of my life would be delightful. At ninety-six, you had lived well, laughing often and loving very much.

"My mother was always so disappointed in me," you shared during our very first visit. "She was a gifted seamstress, known for her buttonholes. She was so proud of her darn buttonholes," you said, rolling your eyes like a teenager. You were your mother's only daughter. "It was so important to her that I learned to make those terrible buttonholes."

"Did you ever learn?"

"No, of course not. I hated buttonholes. Still do."

I asked the next obvious question, "What did you want to do instead?"

You paused, tilted your head, and raised your chin before speaking: "Fly."

I learned that at age twenty-one, with a bit of help from your father, you had earned your pilot's license and that "never did please Mother." As we sat in your front room under your large sun-filled window, your zest for life and sense of adventure were clearly still with you. Your face was filled with wonder and joy as we sat on your couch and talked about the "unimaginable beauty of butterfly metamorphosis."

Flight, no matter who or what creature did it, delighted you. With great detail you shared your flying adventures. Hugging the rim of a great canyon was at the top of your list. You seemed to have an extraordinary relationship with the wild blue yonder. You spent time with the sky each day, carefully positioning your bed and favorite chair to be in full view of it.

Your husband, also a pilot, had died of cancer at a young age, leaving you a single mother of three in the early 1960s. Over the next fifty years, you buried both parents, all your siblings, and a second husband. You had also outlived your circle of friends.

"The sky never leaves" ended every grieving memory you shared with me. "It was the first thing I fell in love with, and we've been together ever since," you said, flashing your brilliant blue eyes and well-worn smile.

A few months before you died, during my regular Friday afternoon visit (I always tried to end my week on a high note), you called out from the bathroom, having excused yourself to "use the facilities." Today, it seemed, you couldn't quite lift yourself back up off the toilet and called for help. "Could you help me? I don't want to waste any more of our visit trying to launch myself."

I entered the bathroom and handed you a towel to cover yourself. You let it drop to the floor. "Oh, honey, at my age, no one has any modesty left. Just hand me another pad from under the sink." I laughed a little and did as I was told. As you finished up, you caught a glimpse of yourself in the wide bathroom mirror. You hesitated, then doubled over in laughter, grabbing the wall behind you and the vanity top.

"Who is that old woman?" You said in hysterics. "What a trip *this* is!"

Your laughter was genuine and infectious, and we got the giggles. It happens to the best of us: one person laughs, and it just goes on and on. You can't stop. The harder you try, the harder it is. We'd settle down and then start giggling again until our faces hurt. It was a joyous infection.

On the surface, we were two women with a walker in a tiny bathroom, trying to accomplish a simple task without knocking each other over. The more profound truth was that your total acceptance of the situation opened the door for joy to enter. It was euphoric.

As the weeks passed, you became frailer. You spoke more frequently about the father of your children and your parents. You often repeated the story of your canyon rim flight. Your children returned from faraway places. Your daughter took you to the beach one last time. Your daughter-in-law filled your apartment with gorgeous orchids. Your sons looked at photo albums with you. There was no unfinished business, no pain, and very little sorrow.

One morning as you awoke under your beloved sky, you collapsed getting out of bed. You waited a little while, but when the time was right you peacefully let go.

In that grace-filled moment, we all knew you were anxious to get your wings.

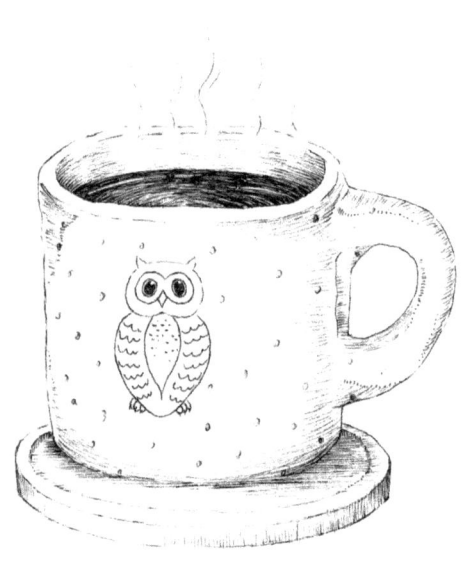

HOT COFFEE

For ninety-nine years, you took pleasure in the simple things. As an only child and a widowed war bride, you found your place in the world later in life. Working as a schoolteacher, you fell in love again, but he passed after his own cancer battle.

Alone for most of your life, you found joy in "good friends and good hair," you'd say with a smirk. Your hairdresser of forty-some-odd years was now your guardian and held your Durable Power of Attorney. You openly questioned why you were the one left behind. All your family, both husbands, and close friends were gone. Most had died long ago.

Sitting in your La-Z-Boy, you loved to watch the birds. Every day the drama unfolded as the neighborhood crows and sparrows gorged themselves on the well-stocked feeder outside your window.

Three times a month, for almost a year, you

and I sat together. We watched the birds and an occasional squirrel jockey for position. But the real highlight of your day, your "reason for living," was "the coffee." You liked it black, and you liked it hot.

"You have to find joy in the small things," you said each time the caregiver handed you a fresh cup. "If I get tired of the coffee, I know it'll be time to die. I don't know if they have coffee in heaven, so I'm going to drink all I can before I go." You took a careful mouthful, holding the hot liquid behind your pursed lips. You paused and savored the feeling of the warm, bitter liquid in your mouth before swallowing it slow and hard. It was your daily ritual, delightfully performed.

The stained speckled-owl mug perfectly fit your cold hands. Its steam circled your nose as if offering its own gratitude for being so well-loved. The love affair seemed mutual.

Your body only lasted two days without your coffee. You went to bed, too tired to get up, and the next evening you died alone in your sleep.

The speckled-owl mug still hung on its hook in the kitchen. I'm not sure when, or if, the staff ever took it down.

√⁄

Some mornings, when my own well-loved mug is warm in my hands, I think about you. Being human can be overwhelming sometimes. It's easy to get caught up and distracted by the emotions and grief in life, but you will always be my gentle reminder to stop and savor the hot coffee.

UNCLE

About sixty years after the handsome high school basketball star married the wholesomely adorable County Fair Beauty Queen, I knocked on your front door.

A live-in caregiver graciously welcomed me and escorted me upstairs. Your wife, just as adorable and beautiful as she once was, delighted in telling me the story of how you met. She giggled, thinking of your persistence, as she "already had several gentleman callers."

Your own eyes twinkled, listening to her retell the story of your courtship, marriage, and rainy honeymoon. You raised two girls together and delighted in every one of your grandchildren. Later, you had two great-grandchildren who found their place among the endless cousins and nearby relatives. You were, indeed, everyone's favorite uncle.

My subsequent visits were very much like the first, as the two of you readily participated in a life review, sharing fantastic tales of family history and wild Italian ancestors. The topic of Italy, and your mother's side of the family, gave me the first glimpse of your softer, less patriarchal side.

You regretted not returning to Italy, walking the town that held your roots and paying your respects to the family vineyard's fertile soil. I saw the grief and regret you were burdening yourself with.

With your permission, I pulled the iPad from my bag. "Show me," I said, typing in the name of the small town in Italy's Graian Alps. The "Street View" in Google Maps came into focus. You were in disbelief.

Together we virtually strolled the streets, finding the town square, a stone fence made by your grandfather, and an iron gate you once climbed. You found the small schoolhouse and the church at the end of a narrow road. It was a trip of a lifetime, summoned by your own index finger. The following week you purchased your own iPad, and your world expanded again.

In time, you became more open and vulnerable with your grief. You worried about your wife, you worried about your family, and apparently, you worried about me, too. You had noticed I wasn't wearing a wedding ring and never spoke of my own children or family. You didn't understand why "a nice girl" like me wasn't married and "taken care of."

As the months passed, you berated me over my lack of a wedding ring, and I badgered you over your love of a certain twenty-four-hour news channel.

"After eighty-seven years of success, community, and witnessed human decency, how could you continually believe a doom and gloom narrative?" I challenged.

"Why are you choosing not to be married and taken care of?" you countered.

The two of us went round and round as "the world was going to hell in a handbag." Your wife found our never-ending banter delightfully entertaining.

Two years into your hospice admission, I stopped by on a Saturday afternoon to celebrate the release of a wine named in your honor from a family member's winery. I introduced you to the man I now share my life with. I believe it took you one firm handshake and several seconds of sustained eye contact before you felt I was sufficiently "taken care of."

As your strong and stable body continually betrayed you with its decline, you (finally) replaced your TV news shows with jigsaw puzzles. Your tinkering mind and spirit found solace in solving the odd shapes and color problems.

One month before you died, you allowed me to join you in your anger. Your failing respiratory system was difficult for a man like you who had always been athletic and stoic. Your physical dependence on others was not an easy hurdle. We talked about your lungs. We thanked your knees for their eight decades of moving you forward. We thanked your strong bridge-playing mind and your orchard-walking big feet. We talked about the legacy of nicotine.

With acceptance, then forgiveness, and then gratitude, you began your goodbyes. The last time we spoke was on the phone. You told me you loved me, and I asked if I could see you the following week. When we hung up the phone, I knew that you weren't so sure.

I did get to see you again. You were asleep in your bed. In all our years together, I had never seen you unshaven or in bedclothes. I knew it was good-bye. I squeezed your hand and hugged your wife. With both of your adult daughters at your bedside, I, too, professed my love.

You died the next day with your wife, your two daughters, and your sweet dog holding vigil.

Almost one year later, after your beauty queen wife had died in your daughter's home, I was invited to your shared memorial service. It was a beautiful day in my favorite cemetery, high on a hill over-looking the Pacific Ocean. Most of your big Italian family was present.

Graveside, relative after relative came up to me and said the same thing: "Oh, *you're* Carolyn! It's so nice to finally meet you! Did you know Uncle always had his shower aide come before your visits?"

"No," I said, confused the first time I heard it. I became increasingly mortified by the fifteenth encounter, knowing full well what would be said next.

"Yeah, Uncle—he always did like the pretty girls."

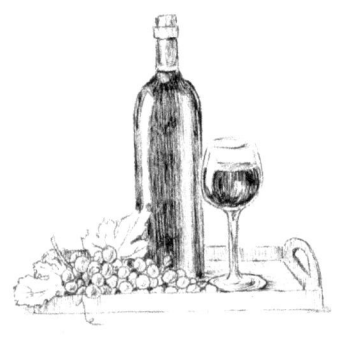

٧/

May you rest in peace, dear Uncle. It was an honor to be one of your girls. Now we both know I will always be taken care of. Cin Cin!

THE GREAT MOTHER TREE

When a redwood dies or is cut down, the tree sends her stored nutrients out through her root system to the circle of children, or burls, surrounding her trunk. Through your front window, I saw your adult children encircling you. It was not lost on me that I was witness to the loving absorption of your nutrients. I knocked softly.

Your busy yard was full of birdbaths, wind chimes, and garden gnomes, so I was not surprised to find each horizontal surface inside covered with generations of art projects, clay handprints, and various treasured collections. Your kitchen was painted a happy yellow, and despite the presence of death in the home, the potted plants exuded life.

On my first, and what would be my only visit, you had called a family meeting. I took my place on one of the sofas across from where you sat in your recliner. Family members filled in the remaining seating, and it felt like everyone had their usual, or perhaps assigned, seat.

Looking at you, fully dressed but reclined in your chair, you were undoubtedly the Great Mother Tree. Your four children widened the circle around you with fifteen grandchildren, who widened it further with twelve great-grandchildren. Two great-great-grandchildren were not present, but their pictures covered the coffee table. Your legacy glowed.

You spoke first, and "the meeting" quickly came to order. As a "Christian woman," you were confident and "knew" where you were going. Your only expressed concern was how you would get there. You did not want to suffer, nor did you want your death to be painful for you or your family. The hospice nurse had already visited, but you were open about your concerns beyond comfort medications and disease processes. You wanted reassurances from Jesus, from God, and the Holy Spirit.

Your adult children wanted to know how to help and what to do. Death was new to you and to them.

I gently asked if God had taken care of you during your eighty-seven years of life. You praised your extended family and confidently implied that He had. "Then why do you think He would stop caring for you in your death?" I asked carefully.

You were quiet as if allowing yourself to answer my question from a deeper place. You smiled at me, and I knew I had provided you with peace. I smiled back.

Knowing your large family was one of the cornerstones of your well-lived life, I offered one of my favorite metaphors to your family:

Our bodies are made to come into this world, and they are made to leave it. As you well know, birth is a miracle. What if death is the same door, just used in a different direction? Much like the birthing process, there is a deathing process. There can be fear of the unknown, agitation, and discomfort. It can be hard work, or labor, to bring a soul into this world, and there can be labor involved in birthing you out. You can read all the books you want on childbirth and talk to other mothers, but at the end of the day, your body will do what it will do. Birth and death are already in your bones. Some people schedule C-Sections or numb themselves to take the edge off, and some choose to feel nothing at all. Others give birth in a field or a swimming pool. There is no right or wrong way to give birth. And there is no right or wrong way to die. As I look around this room, I see you are already surrounded by a room full of caring, loving midwives. You can fight death or be fully present for it, but the outcome will be the same. Like all births, your death will also be a natural rite of passage.

I did not see you again, and I wasn't invited back for another family meeting. There was no need. Your family knew how to midwife, and you knew how to trust your body.

One month later, with generations of midwives surrounding you, your body contracted a few times, you took some panting breaths, and you let go.

\'/

Like the great mother trees deep in the forest, your future generations will exist independent of you above ground. But underneath it, each one will continue to draw sustenance from the root system and the nutrients you so carefully wove below them.

Your roots, Dear Mother, will forever remain intact.

PORCH ROCKS

In celebration of your one-hundredth birthday, a local art museum created an exhibition to showcase your Chinese brush paintings. The talent emerged from your many extended visits to China with your husband. After his death, now more than two decades ago, the brush paintings had become your sanctuary.

I met you in your beautiful Asian art-filled home a year after your exhibition. You were no longer eating food. You told me, "I only eat ice cream." Your smile told me all that I needed to know. The live-in caregivers were well accustomed to making milkshakes for breakfast and milkshakes for lunch. Dinner was usually two small scoops of chocolate. Only recently had you given up the sprinkles and whipped cream.

You were a lifelong learner who had become a schoolteacher, "just as the war was starting and

Judy Garland found Oz," you said, as if still in an overcrowded classroom. You willingly shared your passions for the arts, good ice cream, long hikes, and massive dogs.

The stairs leading up to your front door had piles of rocks and stones collected from long ago hikes and far away vacations. You said they were reminders of your "encounters with the beyond." Sketchpads and tiny glass bottles, each with their special brushes, surrounded you. It was easy to see your creative joy.

"My spirit has not aged; only my body has," you would say. "I used to be young and beautiful. Now I'm just *beautiful*." And you were right.

You knew your body had created itself, and you knew it was fading away. I saw it, too. We all did. You began to withdraw.

As the acceptance of "Yes, I am dying" becomes real, we humans retreat inside ourselves. We sleep more. We talk less. We start spending more time within.

The milkshake meals became small sips rather than slurps. Your body didn't need or want the calories. It's usually the meat or protein our bodies lose interest in first, then the crunchy vegetables or other fiber-rich foods that are harder to digest. Sugar seems to be the "nutrient" we hang on to the longest, although your ice cream soon became more about comfort than sustenance.

The next time I saw you, you were on the couch surrounded by pillows and warm blankets. The chair and well-loved art easel across the room were empty. I asked about the blank pages, but you were happily disoriented in your warm nest. I knew you were enjoying your time a little bit here and a little bit somewhere else.

As your eyes looked past me, I wondered if you saw something I could not witness but wanted to.

The caregivers were concerned about you picking at your clothes and smock sleeves. There seems to be some need to keep our fingers busy as we separate. I brought you a "fidget blanket" with lots of colors, textures, and notions, but your fingers wanted nothing to do with it. I laughed when the caregiver said the mismatched colors were not beautiful enough for you.

Your son was by your side as your skin became clammy and flushed. Your fingernails and hands had death's usual purplish hue. I figured your feet and knees were probably blotchy, too.

After 101 years of pumping, your heart was having trouble maintaining its normal lub-dub rhythm. I silently thanked it for its hard work. That muscle, still beating in your chest, had taken you many places and loved many people. It felt right to thank it for its years of service, despite its current inefficiencies.

Your son and I talked about breathing changes. You were taking long deep breaths followed by a few quick, shallow ones. He knew you might start to sound congested or make some rattling sounds. The hospice nurse had already told him it was your time to go. He stayed close and held your hand.

I never encourage people to stimulate our human senses with music or other distractions during the deathing process. The voices of loved ones always seem to be the most comforting. "They say hearing is the last sense to go, so keep talking to her," I said. "She can hear you even if she can't respond."

The day before you died, your son told me you had a burst of energy and spoke clearly to him. He tearfully shared the memory. He was blessed to be near you and to have the opportunity to thank you for being his mom. As your glassy eyes half opened and you took your last few breaths several minutes apart, your son stayed by your side until your separation was complete and your physical body was empty. He said it was a gift.

One last time after you died, I met with your son. He was packing up your beautiful picture books and artwork from faraway places. The dining room table was covered with valuable collectibles, and he generously asked me if I wanted anything. I did.

\ı,

The eggplant-sized old gray rock from the sunni-
est corner of your front porch sits in my garden.
It reminds my young spirit to stay *beautiful* as my
body encounters the beyond.

IN JEOPARDY

The last time I saw you, I was masked and wearing a yellow plastic gown and blue latex gloves. You were frightened, and I was grief-stricken.

For fourteen months, we'd spent hours in your well-appointed room. You eagerly shared the loving details of each handmade quilt, crayon drawing, and 1970s vacation photo. You always greeted me with a warm and welcoming smile. Unless, of course, it was 12:30. Every day at 12:30 (and again at 5:30), your door closed. Everyone in the board-and-care home stayed away during *Jeopardy!* You knew every contestant and almost every answer. After nine full decades of life, you remained sharp-witted. Alex Trebek had become your good friend. He was a steady engaging presence in your ever-shrinking world.

You had always loved politics and spent many

years volunteering for your favorite candidates. An avid reader, you were proud of making up your own mind on issues after studying independent sources. As a young teen, you volunteered for Herbert Hoover's campaign. After stuffing envelopes for hours with your mother, you still remembered the disappointment of being too young to vote.

In your ninety-ninth year of life, you bargained with God to let you live long enough to vote in the upcoming presidential election. The day your absentee ballot arrived, you read every word and savored each black ink-filled oval. It would be the last day I saw your joy.

When Alex Trebek lost his life to pancreatic cancer a few days after the presidential election winner was announced, you sobbed for both man and country.

We talked about the friends you had lost to cancer. We talked about your husband's death, too, and how the most-challenging part was still falling asleep each night. For sixty-five years, your head had rested peacefully on his chest, his arms folded tenderly around you. "Now, every night is cold and lonely," you said. I deeply listened to the longings for what had been—and what would never be again.

Your weary heart was having trouble keeping up. You were getting more confused, and you knew it. The change would be another isolating loss.

I increased my visits to see you more often. You liked to hold my hand and reached for it each time I arrived. Together, we honored your sadness and held your grief. We looked at photographs and talked about happy memories and goodnight sleeps. The routine brought you some clarity and an occasional weary smile.

The multiple losses had taken their toll on your will to live. You questioned why you were still here, why you were the one left behind. "Why doesn't God want me?"

On your 100th birthday, you asked God if it was enough. It would not be.

On your 101st birthday, despite your dementia,

you remembered to ask God again.

On your 102nd birthday, we gathered around your bed and sang to you. You cried and said you wanted to go home.

Two months before your 103rd birthday, the world shut down because of COVID-19. Board-and-care facilities, convalescent homes, hospitals, and private homes all locked their doors to outside visitors.

I tried to see you through a window. I cheerfully waved and smiled, eager to maintain my connection with you, but you didn't smile back. I was told you didn't understand why I wouldn't come inside. You fretted as if you'd done something wrong and had hurt my feelings. You asked the caregiver why I was mad at you. My well-meaning window visit had caused more confusion than connection. The caregiver asked me not to return.

You weren't the only patient I lost when the world shut down. The connection I had with all thirty-six of my patients was lost. The medicine

I provided could not be administered through a pane of glass or telephone line, and I could not comfort the dying in a Zoom meeting.

Once hospice staff members were deemed "essential," we were re-issued Personal Protective Equipment (PPE). The gowns, gloves, and face shields usually reserved for infectious-disease patients became protocol. Cone-shaped N-95 masks, daily temperature checks, and weekly Health Department nose swabs were now mandatory.

When a few doors opened, I became a much-needed cellphone holder as spouses and family members gathered for heartbreaking FaceTime goodbyes. My once-warm hands were now covered in cold latex gloves. My warm smile and soft, comforting voice were now muffled by a barrier of molded polypropylene fibers held by a tight elastic band. I did the best I could to keep a warm human connection. I never wanted death to feel like a medical event.

✳

The last time I saw you, I was masked, with a yellow plastic gown and blue latex gloves. You pulled away from me, and there was nothing I could do about the fright in your eyes. The health protocols had broken our connection. I slowly backed away. I didn't want to make it worse. I melted back into the hallway, defeated. I would never see you again.

My heart ached for you and for our world.

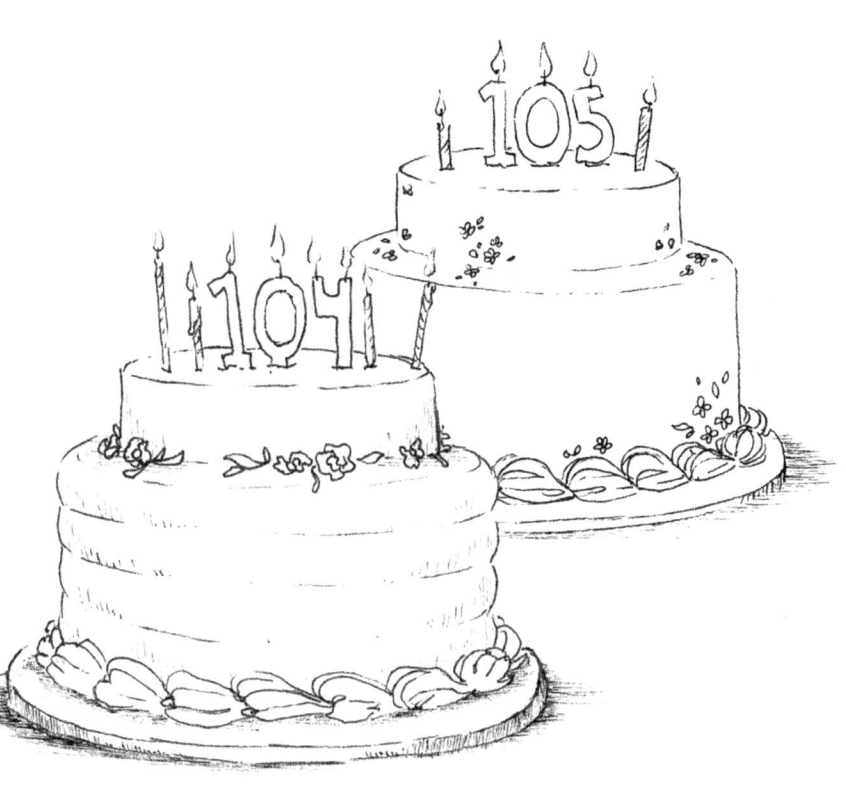

. . . 104th birthday . . . 105th birthday. . .

LET'S GO FOR A WALK

Walking up to your front door for the first time, I paused to smell the Cecile Brunner climbing rosebush intertwined with your front porch. It is my mother's favorite, and I can't pass one without hearing her say, "Take time to smell the roses." As the well-loved devoted daughter, I stopped and buried my nose, inhaling deeply. It was Valentine's Day, and my nose was buried in a beautiful pink rose. I smiled.

I knocked on your door and noticed the stone dog statue. Dog people. I smiled again. When the door opened, I was greeted with the familiar face of unyielding fatigue. The caring spouse who can no longer "just be" the husband or the wife but has become the full-time caregiver. I saw it in your eyes. You would do anything for your wife, and you had exhausted yourself trying.

We sat at your kitchen table overlooking the lake and a familiar mountain. You shared stories about a Panama deployment and a carefully crafted pink suit, but it was not the life stories that touched me. It was the way your wife looked at you. Between her now-shallow breaths, there was endearment, love, respect, and partnership. In you, she found her comfort and her peace. You two are a love story.

On my next visit, I encouraged you to take a walk. "Take a few minutes to yourself," I said. "I will hold her close and safe." When you returned, a little light was back in your eyes. The three of us only sat at your kitchen table three times. After sixty-seven years of marriage and during her eighty-seventh trip around the sun, your wife took her last soft breath. She was ready, but I wasn't sure you were.

Your care team was worried about you. We flagged you as "moderate risk" for our bereavement team. You were stoic and not one to ask for help, let alone support. Knowing that using the telephone was difficult for your eighty-eight-year-old ears, I sent an email. "Would you like to go for a walk?"

And so it began.

Mid-pandemic, when only the outdoors was safe, and the world was on hold, we walked. And we walked again. I not only learned about your grief for your wife but also for your daughter, who had lost her battles with disease and life too young. I learned about your love of photography, tennis, and philosophies, but not religions. I learned of your devotion to purpose.

You learned that I was suffering from compassion fatigue, that the work was getting harder and heavier. In the grief, I struggled to keep home, work, and mind balanced in the rapidly changing world outside our walks.

We meandered on to the path of poetry. I shared Mary Oliver. You got brave and started to write your own, which I share here with your permission:

The Walk

Today I am walking in search of Heaven,
Looking for the Lady that I call my Soulmate
I lost her, but I will find her once again
When I find her, I will give her a big hug,
And an even bigger kiss
And then we will walk on,

The rest of the way,
Together once again …

Dick Bray, of "Pat and Dick"

Then I got brave and wrote this book with (and for) you.

The act of walking was a healing time for us. The circles made on that middle school track changed you. They changed me, too. Your words have stopped me in my tracks more than once.

Our walks have become hikes, which have become pilgrimages into the woods and out of our less-forgiving minds. We have shared a labyrinth of possibilities. When the world allowed it, we returned to your kitchen table, still overlooking the lake and familiar mountain, but we no longer talk of Panama or pink suits.

Now we write and talk about the...

Words of Life:

Faith and Love,
Grace and Beauty,
Anger and Happiness.

Words of Life,
Words of Freedom,
Words of Being....

... and I intend to walk you home, too.

THE CANDYMAN

I grew up in an affluent suburb of Washington, D.C.. The National Mall and Vietnam Veterans Memorial were frequent stops when friends and family visited. In contrast to the white Lincoln Memorial and other national monuments, the Vietnam Veterans Memorial is a huge 400-foot wall of black granite sunken into the earth. There are 58,000 names—each one carefully etched into the stone. Standing at the base of the dark monument was the first time in my early life I witnessed grief.

The intimidating wall that made men cry mystified me. As a kid, I had no context to understand the grief I witnessed each time we visited. Later, when a high school friend was killed in an automobile accident, I watched his little sister run back to his coffin before being scooped up by my friend's dad. I recognized the look on their faces from the black granite wall. Death scared me.

As a young adult I avoided every cemetery and every war movie. They made me uncomfortable. My avoidance and discomfort felt like a character flaw. I couldn't explain it, but I felt it. Then one weekday afternoon through my television set Oprah spoke to me: "People fear what they do not understand." It was my own *aha moment.*

The next day, I signed up to become a hospice volunteer. The weekly trainings taught me to be a good listener. They taught me to hold the tension of sadness and grief without trying to fix it. The teachers changed my perceptions of what it meant to die and what it meant to grieve. Oprah was right—my fear began to transform.

My first assignment was to provide "respite" for a male patient being cared for by his brother. With curiosity and an open heart, I arrived at their small home tucked into the woods. My patient's brother was warm and welcoming. He walked me into the bedroom and introduced me to his brother, who looked perfectly healthy. He was just a guy in his pajamas ready to take a nap.

I sat in his room chatting, offering social dialogue, and asking lots of questions. My hospice volunteer training had encouraged me to listen more than speak. We discovered that we both loved candy bars and discussed in detail the pros and cons of various bars. We made each other laugh.

After my second visit, I got into my car and noticed something on my windshield. I got out and lifted the windshield wiper. Wrapped in a paper towel was a candy bar. I laughed and knew I had made a new friend. As the months went by, I visited this patient and his brother weekly. Each time I returned to my car, a new candy bar was tucked under the wiper. With great fanfare they always denied knowing anything about it.

As my newfound Candyman declined, our conversations became fewer and fewer. I sat at his bedside, sometimes reading him the newspaper, sometimes just holding his hand. My time there became less about the "doing" and more about the "being." Our backgrounds were very different, and our values and beliefs were different too, but we enjoyed our friendship almost as much as we enjoyed the candy bars.

The grief I witnessed each time I visited the Vietnam Veterans Memorial returned to my mind as I drove down the narrow road to his wooded home on what I knew was my last visit. I felt sad and silently wondered if his name would be etched in stone somewhere sacred, too.

I knocked on the door and was greeted unexpectedly by a woman. The extended family I had never seen or heard of had arrived, and my friend now slept in a hospital bed. The bed had been moved to the center of the living room, loud Gospel music playing from the TV. The day was an intimate time for his family. They were losing a family member. No one in the room knew anything about me, my economic status, my education, my faith—none of it mattered. In life, we didn't have much in common, but in this man's death, we shared a common grace.

The plastic hospice volunteer name badge around my neck had granted me entrance to a whole new world. It was a new way of seeing people. It was a new way of being. On the outside, we were different. On the inside, we were the same.

Before I left, I squeezed my new friend's hand and kissed him on the forehead. His brow was hot. He seemed to be a little bit here and a little bit somewhere else. His uneven breathing was wet and labored. His hands looked mottled. I leaned forward again and paused with my lips on his warm forehead. I closed my eyes and silently thanked him for allowing me into his home. I knew in my heart that this exact moment would always be with me. This man, this space, this feeling would never leave.

The Candyman died in the fall of 1998, his brother and family at his side.

༈

The experience of becoming a hospice volunteer changed my life. Learning all I could about my fears, and where they had come from, led me to my life's work.

SACRED HEART

Twenty-three years later, and twenty-five hundred miles to the west of the woods where the Candyman died, I find myself now sitting at your bedside. I am no longer a well-trained hospice volunteer, but a well-worn hospice spiritual counselor.

You are comfortable in this beautiful room with high ceilings, wood floors, and breathtaking vineyard views. You are impeccably cared for. Your room is quiet and still, and you look beautifully at peace.

I did not arrive at your bedside emotionally clean. I still carry this morning's grief from a spouse whose husband of fifty-four years no longer recognizes her. The life review, compassionate listening, and deep questioning from the afternoon's three home visits are in me, too. I can't seem to shake them. The obligation of training the new staff member I was with when your family called is still with me.

Then there are my responsibilities at home waiting for me and already requiring some attention. I have carried all of this with me into your room today, knowing full well it doesn't belong here. Knowing this, and feeling guilty about it, further keeps me from being fully present with you.

Sitting here, in this room, in your quiet sacred space, I force myself to focus on my breath. I fully inhale and mindfully let the breath go, feeling the air move in and out of my now familiar N-95 mask. I melt into the sky-blue upholstered chair at your bedside. As the chair and presence support me, I am overcome by my own need for quiet sanctuary.

I allow myself to feel what I have known for some time. I am beyond compassion fatigue. I am exhausted to the point of burnout. Silent tears descend on my cheek. I lean further into the grace as you sleep peacefully before me.

"I am so sorry," I whisper. My muffled voice cracks, "I am so tired, and you look so beautiful."

You remain unresponsive.

Less than an hour ago the text came. Could I sit with a newly admitted patient? A woman was dying. The family was on their way from Los Angeles, and they did not want her to die alone. Could I go?

How could I not? You were dying.

Now I am here, at your bedside. You are resting with your fingers loosely clasped together. Your hair is soft and wispy around your relaxed face, and your breath is shallow.

In the stillness, I offer a blessing to your family, knowing they are rushing to return to your side. I have never met or spoken to them. I have never met or spoken to you, but here we are together—you and I— waiting quietly for their arrival and your departure.

We are silent together, my breath intentionally mindful of yours as I struggle to bring my whole self to you again. Twenty, maybe thirty breaths, we stay still together in this sacred thin place between our two worlds.

I am again overcome by my feelings of gratitude, fatigue, and grief that well up inside my weary heart. The voice in my mind continues to ask my heart how much longer I can do this work. My heart doesn't answer, or maybe I just keep refusing to listen.

I bow my head in reverence to you, and truth be told, in reverence to all those who have gone before you: the Uncle, the Woman Who Loved the Sky, and Ms. Orange Tree. The Amplified Pain and the Bass Fisherman are here. All our ancestors—yours and mine—are in this thin sacred space. How could they not be?

I reach over and gently place my hand on one of yours. You open your foggy eyes. We look at each other for the first time, although I have already felt seen. I smile and squeeze your hand. I nod and thank you for allowing me to be in this holy enclosure with you. You gently close your eyes and return to stillness.

In the silence, you slowly pull my hand over your ribcage. You place my hand over your own heart—and rest it there.

Instantly, I am flooded with a warm feeling of permission.

I see myself in a room seated among a circle of occupied wooden chairs. I stand up, bow, and step backward, removing myself from the circle. I move to the back wall of the small fire-lit room and stand among the others, facing the work, but no longer in it. The vision fades.

I am released.

I stay in this grace with you until your loving family arrives. I tell them how special you are. They nod in full agreement. I lean forward and press my lips to the back of your hand. I thank you for the privilege of sitting with you. Hugs and gentle tears are exchanged in your honor. Before leaving your space, I turn in the doorway and bow slightly towards you. My heart bows to yours.

As I slowly walk outside, and back into the doing world, I know this exact moment will always be with me. This woman, this space, this feeling will never leave.

٭

The next night, surrounded by your loving family, you die peacefully in your sleep. A few miles further west, I fall asleep with a smile on my face. We are both free.

TRANSITIONS

For many years I had the privilege of sitting with the sad, the mad, and the scared. I also sat with the confused and the grateful. Every day the dying let me into their homes; most let me into their hearts. Each day I had an opportunity to make a difference, and each visit could be filled with meaning and purpose. And yet, day after day, death after death, carrying that privilege left a mark. When the work that had invited me in gave me permission to leave, I listened and handed in my notice.

Leaving my patients was harrowing; they usually left me behind. Now I was the one letting go without really knowing what was next. With an important part of my life coming to an end, I was the one in need of spiritual counseling. Instead of sitting with the physically dying, I began to sit with my own transition. I went inside to the dark places and questioned my thoughts. Without judgment,

I held the tension between my grief and freedom. I questioned the stories I told myself about work, money, and responsibility. I wondered what was true. I was present in the sacred thin place between my two worlds. My hospice experience had taught me the value of feeling *all* the feelings. The only way out of my dark thoughts was through them.

٭

Walking out of the hospice office that last Friday afternoon, I looked down at the ground. There, at my feet, was a single white feather. I picked it up and twirled it between my fingers. Amused, I looked up to the sky.

"It was a privilege," I whispered. As I bowed my head and leaned further into the grace.

Two months later, on a dark foggy morning, I lit a candle and curled up in my favorite overstuffed chair. Gripping my hot coffee I longed for the warmth of end-of-life friendships. It didn't matter if the dying were dirty or clean, wealthy or poor, atheist or evangelical. I loved the humanity of them all. I longed to sit with the fearful and the free. Now, my love had nowhere to go.

For each of my patients I had kept a single sheet of notebook paper where I logged antiquated notes and personal quips, no longer welcome in the world of electronic medical records. The pages had no real names or identifying information, only nicknames to help me differentiate between all the Johns, Roberts, and Marys I'd been assigned over the years.

Still in my pajamas, I returned to my two-foot stack of archives and found patient number one. I read my notes...and I remembered. I remembered who the Sock Monkey was. I could picture her room and what she was wearing. I remembered the cold.

I gifted myself the time to once again grieve

her loss and acknowledge my own. I wanted to tell her she was not forgotten, so I wrote her a letter.

My new morning ritual continued for months. Each page, each memory, each feeling was set free. It was a joy to spend time with these people again. Some got dissertations, some got sticky notes. A handful got, "Oh, no! I don't want to spend another minute with you."

Some notes made me laugh. Others made me cry. I allowed myself the time and space to remember the hands I had held and acknowledge how those dying hands continue to hold me.

☆

Perhaps in these pages they have held you too.

A GLORIOUS MESS

This being human is such a glorious mess. The ups and downs of life and finally the ups and downs of death. If there is one lesson I have learned from the dying, it is this: we humans tend to die the way we live. I have seen it over and over again.

If you know how to be happy in your life, you will know how to die with a smile on your face. If you are anxious in life, you will worry your way to death. If you spend time being angry in life, you will waste a lot of time being angry at death, too. If you love drama or being the center of attention in life, don't worry; your death will be full of great drama as everyone around you tries to meet your needs (and your wants).

Participating in the end-of-life journey tends to make each of us, dying or not, more of who we already are. Friends and family who are open, loving, and caring tend to become even more of those things. If a sibling or spouse is scared and fearful, they tend to become so scared the fear often shows up as anger or even control. Those who focus on money, or other resources like food and medications, tend to become even more focused on those things. That's why there are so many stories of family tensions and dramas playing out during the end of someone's life. The magnifying glass named "running out of time" makes everyone a more exaggerated version of themselves.

Families often asked me why I did this work, and my answer (regardless of who they were or why they were asking) was always the same: I loved this work because it was real. There is a lot less BS to wade through when you meet someone who knows they are dying than in any other circumstance. The dying know there is no cure at the end of life, but they are deeply motivated to heal.

If it is important to you to have a peaceful death, you will need to create a peaceful life. It's not easy, but it's not complicated either. You will die the way you live. We all do.

May we rest in peace.

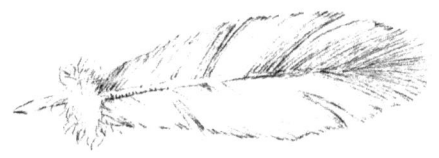

ACKNOWLEDGMENTS

Thank you...

Linda Sherrill, for teaching a "learning-differently" kid like me that I am lovable and capable.

Dr. John Stratton, of then Ashland College, for being the first person on the planet to convince me I could—and should—write.

Sue Carpenter and nurse Dawn of then Monongalia Hospice, in Morgantown, West Virginia, for educating me on life, death, and the important things in between.

Ken, Kenny, Kristi, Stephanie (ASD), and Lindee for teaching me about love and about loss.

Brian Pritt, Luis Sarmiento, Jerry Jordano, and Marc Garcia of Central Coast Home Health and Hospice, in San Luis Obispo, California, for the opportunity and the cardboard box caskets.

Maryhelen Zabas, Richard Groves and the Sacred Art of Living Center, in Bend, Oregon, for the sacred toolbox and lifelong friendships.

My spiritual brother Jay Horn and beloved Rabbi Jayne Simon, for your wisdom and mentoring.

Janet, George, Lou, Mel, Kathleen, Wilma, Pat, Gene, Sofia, Barbara, Julia, Roxanne, Jean, Betsey, Patricia, Vickie, Annabel, David, William, and Sarah, for your guidance in this world and beyond it.

Rick Kerpsack, and then Rita King, and then Mona Taylor, you were right. I needed to write a book.

Joanna Nowinski, for authentically reading it first and for decades of good hair therapy.

Diane Shabazian, Debbie Holly, Mark Sczbecki and Neil Ticktin, for your time, genuine insights, and ongoing friendships.

Angela Ivey and Nathaniel Hansen, for making my voice stronger and better. You are Divine intervention.

Soul sisters Janie Eddleman, Candy Negrete, and Karen Preskenis, for holding me in your hearts and encouraging me with heartfelt wisdom. This book would not have happened without you.

Merci de m'avoir appris des choses sur les crevettes, merci d'être resté fidèle à ma plume et d'avoir aimé mon adorable Pop.

Gary Walker and my gift of a mother, Annie/G Rohrbach-Walker, thank you for your inspiration, insights, encouraging hugs, and life changing trips to the well.

Jack Kornfield, Byron Katie, the Enneagram, and Irish Hills, for bringing me home.

Eldon and Maya, thank you for being a part of me as I hold you close, while learning to let you go. I love you both more than yoga.

And to Drew, thank you for always enhancing my experience, connecting dots I don't always see, and for loving me — exactly the way you do.

www.ingramcontent.com/pod-product-compliance
Lightning Source LLC
Chambersburg PA
CBHW051521120626
46551CB00012B/1030